High Protein, Low Carb Cookbook Recipes for Weight Loss

Simple, Satisfying Recipes with a 30-Day Meal Plan to Burn Fat, Control Hunger, and Lose Weight Without Guesswork

Abigail Douglas

Table of Contents

High Protein, Low Carb Cookbook Recipes for Weight

Loss 1

Preface 15

Introduction 19

Why This Way of Eating Works (Without the Drama)

.... 19

What "High Protein, Low Carb" Really Means (In

Plain Language) 20

Why Protein Supports Fat Loss, Fullness, and Energy

.... 21

Why Lowering Refined Carbs—Not Eliminating

Them—Matters 21

How to Use This Book Day by Day with Confidence

.... 23

Chapter 1 26

The Simple Rules That Guide Every Meal 26

The Protein-First Plate (How to Build Meals

Without Counting) 26

Choosing Carbs Wisely (What Stays, What Goes) 27

Fats That Support Satiety Without Excess 29

Portion Guidance Using Visual Cues (No Scales, No

Apps) 30

How to Shop Once and Eat All Week 31

Why These Rules Work Together 31

.... 33

Chapter 2 34

Your 30-Day Weight Loss Meal Plan (How It's

Structured)... 34

How the 30 Days Are Organized for Ease............. 34

Why Meals Repeat Strategically (Less Thinking,

Better Adherence) 35

How to Swap Meals Without Breaking the Plan ... 36

Eating Out or Busy-Day Adjustments 37

What to Drink During the Plan 38

Why This Structure Works... 39

.... 40

Chapter 3 42

High-Protein Breakfasts (Days 1–30)....................... 42

Why Breakfast Protein Matters for Appetite Control 43

Simple Morning Meals Ready in 5–15 Minutes........ 43

No Powders Required (Protein Comes from Food)... 44

Recipe Types Included 45

   Egg-Based Breakfasts 45

   Greek Yogurt Bowls................................ 46

   Cottage Cheese Plates 46

   Simple Breakfast Scrambles 46

   Make-Ahead Options for Busy Mornings 46

30-Day Breakfast Rotation (Examples)...................... 47

Chapter 4 51

Protein-Focused Lunches for Steady Energy............. 51

How to Build a Filling Lunch Without Bread Overload

.... 52

Packable Lunches for Work or Home 53

Leftover-Friendly Meals 53

Recipe Types Included 54

    Chicken Bowls 54

    Tuna and Salmon Plates 55

    Turkey and Veggie Skillets 55

    Simple Salads with Real Protein............................ 55

Warm Lunch Options for Comfort............................ 56

30-Day Lunch Rotation (Examples)........................... 56

Chapter 5 59

Easy High-Protein Dinners (No Fancy Cooking)...... 59

Why Dinner Doesn't Need to Be Heavy to Be

Satisfying 59

One-Pan and Stovetop Meals.................................... 60

Comfort-Style Dishes Made Lighter.......................... 61

Recipe Types Included 62

Baked Chicken and Fish 62

Beef and Vegetable Skillets 62

Simple Stir-Fries 62

Sheet-Pan Meals.. 63

Slow Evenings, Minimal Cleanup 63

30-Day Dinner Rotation (Examples) 63

Chapter 6 67

Week 1 – Reset and Simplicity 67

Your Full 7-Day Plan (Breakfast, Lunch, Dinner). 67

Grocery List Guidance (Shop Once, Eat All Week) .. 70

What to Expect in the First Week (Hunger, Energy,

Adjustments) 71

Chapter 7 74

Week 2 – Consistency Builds Momentum................. 74

Your Full 7-Day Plan (Week 2) 74

Why Repeating Meals Works (And Why It Matters

Now).. 77

Staying Full Without Snacking 78

Chapter 8 81

Week 3 – Confidence and Rhythm 81

Your Full 7-Day Plan (Week 3) 81

How Appetite Naturally Stabilizes 84

Eating Out Adjustments (If Needed) 85

What This Week Represents 85

Chapter 9 87

Week 4 – Making It Sustainable 87

Your Final 7-Day Plan (Week 4)............................... 87

How to Continue Beyond Day 30 90

Transitioning Into Long-Term Habits 91

What Success Really Looks Like 91

How to Move Forward 92

Chapter 10 94

After the 30 Days – How to Keep the Weight Off 94

How to Repeat the Plan (Without Burnout) 94

When and How to Add Carbs Back Carefully 95

Protein Habits for Long-Term Success 97

Avoiding Rebound Weight Gain 97

What Maintenance Really Means 98

Moving Forward With Confidence 99

Bonus Section 100

Simple Swaps & Emergency Meals........................ 100

Fast Protein Swaps When Ingredients Are Missing 100

10-Minute Emergency Meals.................................... 101

What to Do on High-Stress Days............................ 102

The Real Purpose of This Section........................... 103

Acknowledgment 105

DISCLAIMER

The information in this book is provided for educational and informational purposes only and is not intended as a substitute for professional medical advice, diagnosis, or treatment.

Always seek the advice of your physician, qualified health provider, or registered dietitian with any questions you may have regarding a medical condition, dietary change, or wellness practice.

Never disregard professional medical advice or delay seeking it because of something you have read in this book.

The author and publisher disclaim any liability for any loss or damage arising directly or indirectly from the use of this material.

Every effort has been made to ensure the accuracy of information presented; however, individual results will vary, and readers are encouraged to honor their unique health needs.

Preface

This book was written for people who want weight loss to feel **clear, doable, and grounded** in real life—not overwhelming, experimental, or extreme.

If you've ever felt tired of plans that promise fast results but collapse the moment life gets busy, you're not alone. Most people don't struggle because they lack discipline. They struggle because they're given advice that's too complicated to sustain. Endless rules. Conflicting guidance. Meals that look good on paper but don't fit normal routines.

This **High Protein, Low Carb Cookbook for Weight Loss** was created to solve that exact problem.

The approach in these pages is intentionally straightforward. No calorie counting. No macro tracking. No expensive ingredients. No "detoxes," "resets," or trendy hacks that come and go. Instead, you'll find **simple**

high-protein, low-carb recipes, a clear 30-day meal plan, and practical guidance you can apply immediately—using foods you can buy at any local grocery store.

The focus is on meals that keep you **full, energized, and consistent.** Protein is prioritized because it supports appetite control, helps preserve muscle, and makes weight loss easier to maintain. Carbohydrates are managed—not eliminated—so you can lose weight without feeling deprived. Meals repeat strategically to reduce decision fatigue and make healthy eating automatic rather than effortful.

This is not a crash diet. It's not a challenge with an expiration date. It's a **realistic weight loss plan** designed to fit into everyday life—busy schedules, family dinners, workdays, and unexpected stress included.

Inside, you'll find:

- A **30-day high-protein, low-carb meal plan** with breakfast, lunch, and dinner laid out clearly
- **Easy recipes for weight loss** that require minimal prep and no special equipment
- Simple food rules that remove guesswork and build confidence
- Practical strategies to avoid rebound weight gain after the 30 days
- Emergency meal options for busy or high-stress days

Most importantly, this book is built around sustainability. The goal isn't just to lose weight—it's to understand how to eat in a way that feels calm, satisfying, and repeatable long after the plan ends.

If you follow this approach, you won't just see changes on the scale. You'll gain clarity around food, confidence in your choices, and a structure you can return to whenever life pulls you off track.

That's how weight loss lasts.

Welcome to a simpler way of eating—one that works with your life, not against it.

Introduction

Why This Way of Eating Works (Without the Drama)

Most people don't fail at weight loss because they lack willpower. They fail because they are handed plans that are confusing, extreme, or simply incompatible with real life. Plans that demand perfection. Rules that change every few months. Advice that sounds convincing but collapses the moment stress, hunger, or a busy day shows up.

This book exists to remove that friction.

A high-protein, low-carb way of eating works not because it is trendy or clever, but because it aligns with how the body actually responds to food. It reduces constant hunger. It steadies energy. It makes meals feel satisfying instead of restrictive. And most importantly, it is something you can repeat day after day without mental exhaustion.

There is no drama here—because results don't require it.

What "High Protein, Low Carb" Really Means (In Plain Language)

High protein, low carb does not mean cutting out entire food groups or surviving on shakes and supplements. It simply means this: most of your meals are built around a solid source of protein, while refined, fast-digesting carbohydrates are kept in check.

Protein is the anchor of every plate. Carbohydrates are chosen carefully, not feared. Fats are used reasonably, not exaggerated. Meals look like food you recognize— because they are.

You are not chasing numbers. You are building meals that naturally support appetite control and steady progress.

Why Protein Supports Fat Loss, Fullness, and Energy

Protein does more than any other nutrient to help you feel satisfied after eating. It slows digestion, reduces cravings, and helps preserve lean muscle while weight is coming off. When protein intake is adequate, hunger becomes quieter. Energy becomes steadier. Decision-making around food becomes easier.

This matters because fat loss does not come from eating less and suffering more—it comes from eating in a way that allows consistency. Protein makes that consistency possible.

Why Lowering Refined Carbs—Not Eliminating Them—Matters

The problem is not carbohydrates themselves. The problem is excess refined carbs that digest quickly, spike blood sugar, and leave you hungry again soon after eating.

Breaded foods, sugary snacks, sweet drinks, and highly processed meals make it difficult to regulate appetite.

This plan lowers those foods—not to punish you, but to restore balance. Carbs that come from vegetables, dairy, legumes, and whole foods still have a place. The goal is not zero carbs. The goal is fewer foods that work against you.

What This Plan Is

This plan is simple.

It is structured.

It is realistic.

You will follow a clear 30-day meal plan with breakfast, lunch, and dinner laid out for you. Ingredients are familiar. Cooking methods are straightforward. Meals repeat strategically so you are not constantly relearning how to eat.

This is not a test of discipline. It is a system that removes guesswork.

What This Plan Is Not

This is not a crash diet.

It is not an elimination challenge.

It is not a trend designed to impress on social media.

There are no "detox" promises, no extreme carb bans, no unrealistic timelines. You will not be asked to suffer through hunger, skip meals, or rely on expensive specialty products. If a plan cannot fit into normal life, it does not belong here.

How to Use This Book Day by Day with Confidence

Read once. Follow daily. Repeat as needed.

You do not need to understand nutrition science to succeed with this book. Each day tells you what to eat. Each week builds momentum. If you miss a meal or swap a dish, you simply continue—no restarting required.

Progress comes from repetition, not perfection.

By the end of these 30 days, you will not only see changes in weight—you will understand how to eat in a way that feels stable, satisfying, and sustainable. And that understanding is what makes results last.

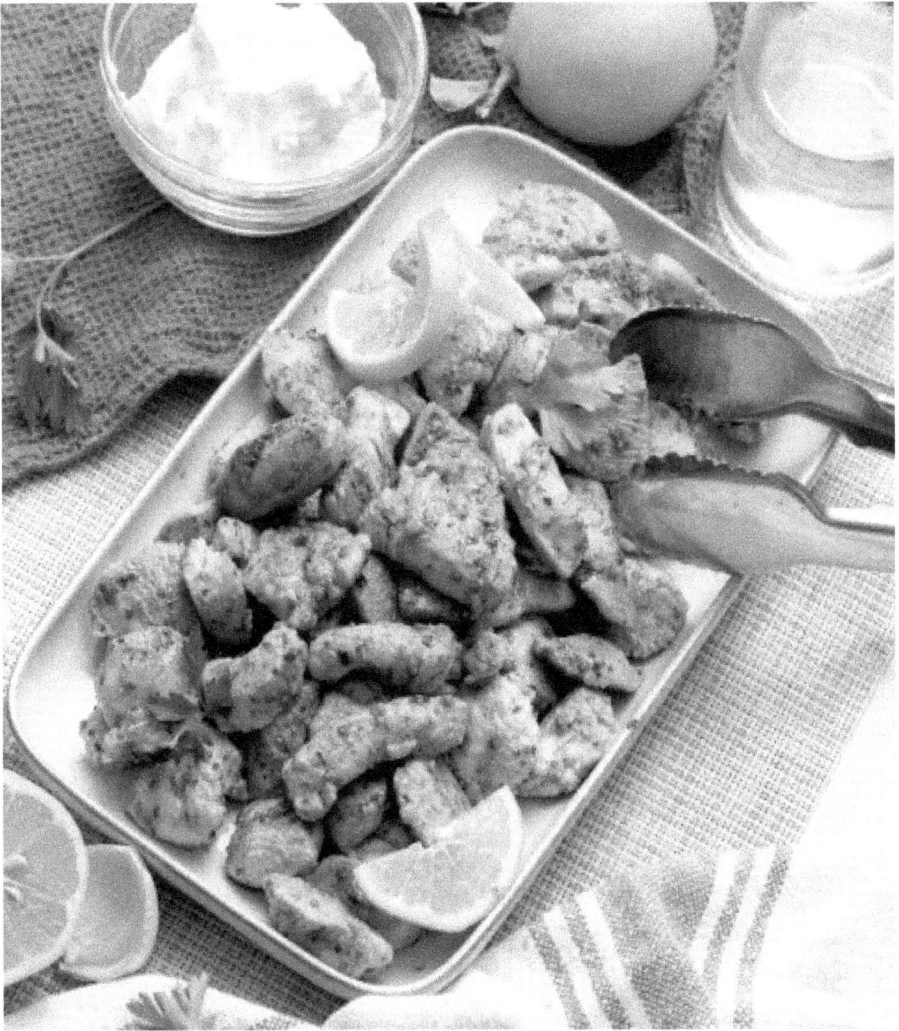

Chapter 1

The Simple Rules That Guide Every Meal

Weight loss becomes complicated when food choices feel like a math problem. Numbers, apps, measurements, rules stacked on rules—eventually, the plan collapses under its own weight. The purpose of this chapter is to strip all of that away and replace it with a few steady principles you can rely on every time you eat.

These rules are not restrictive. They are grounding. Once you understand them, meals stop feeling uncertain—and consistency becomes natural.

The Protein-First Plate (How to Build Meals Without Counting)

Every meal in this book starts with one simple question:

Where is the protein?

Protein is the foundation because it does the most important work. It keeps you full, stabilizes appetite, and helps preserve muscle as weight comes off. When protein leads the plate, everything else falls into place more easily.

A protein-first plate simply means:

- You choose your protein source first
- You build the rest of the meal around it

This could be eggs, chicken, fish, turkey, beef, yogurt, cottage cheese, or other familiar options. No weighing. No tracking. If protein is clearly present and substantial, the meal is doing its job.

If you ever feel unsure about a meal, look at the plate. If protein is missing or just an afterthought, hunger will show up sooner than you want.

Choosing Carbs Wisely (What

Stays, What Goes)

Carbohydrates are not the enemy—but not all carbs work the same way in the body.

This plan focuses on **lowering refined, fast-digesting carbs**, not eliminating carbs entirely. Foods that spike hunger quickly tend to slow progress and make adherence harder. These are the items you'll see less often here.

What stays:

- Vegetables
- Dairy-based carbs like yogurt
- Legumes in modest portions
- Naturally occurring carbs that come with fiber and structure

What goes (or becomes occasional):

- Sugary snacks and drinks
- White bread, pastries, and heavily refined foods

- Meals built mostly around starch with little protein

The goal is calm energy—not spikes and crashes.

Fats That Support Satiety Without Excess

Fat helps food taste good and feel satisfying, but it works best when used intentionally—not heavily.

In this approach, fat:

- Supports fullness
- Adds flavor
- Complements protein

It does not overwhelm the plate.

You'll see fats like olive oil, eggs, dairy, and naturally occurring fats from meats used in reasonable amounts. Enough to feel satisfied. Not so much that calories quietly add up without improving fullness.

When protein leads and carbs are controlled, fat naturally finds its balance.

Portion Guidance Using Visual Cues (No Scales, No Apps)

This book avoids tools that turn eating into a technical exercise. Instead, it relies on visual balance.

A simple visual guideline:

- Protein takes up the largest portion of the plate
- Vegetables fill the rest generously
- Carbs, when included, stay modest
- Fats are present but not dominating

If the plate looks balanced and satisfying, it usually is.

Your appetite is allowed to guide you here. Eat until comfortably full. Stop when satisfied—not stuffed. Over time, your hunger signals will become more reliable.

How to Shop Once and Eat All Week

Consistency gets easier when food decisions are already made.

This plan is built around:

- Repeatable ingredients
- Overlapping meals
- Simple grocery lists

You'll notice the same proteins and vegetables appearing across multiple recipes. This isn't boring—it's efficient. Shopping becomes faster. Cooking becomes easier. And food waste drops dramatically.

When the kitchen is stocked with the right basics, meals stop feeling like a daily challenge.

Why These Rules Work Together

None of these rules work in isolation. Together, they create a system that:

- Reduces hunger
- Simplifies choices
- Encourages repetition
- Fits real life

You don't need to master nutrition. You just need a few rules you can trust.

And now you have them.

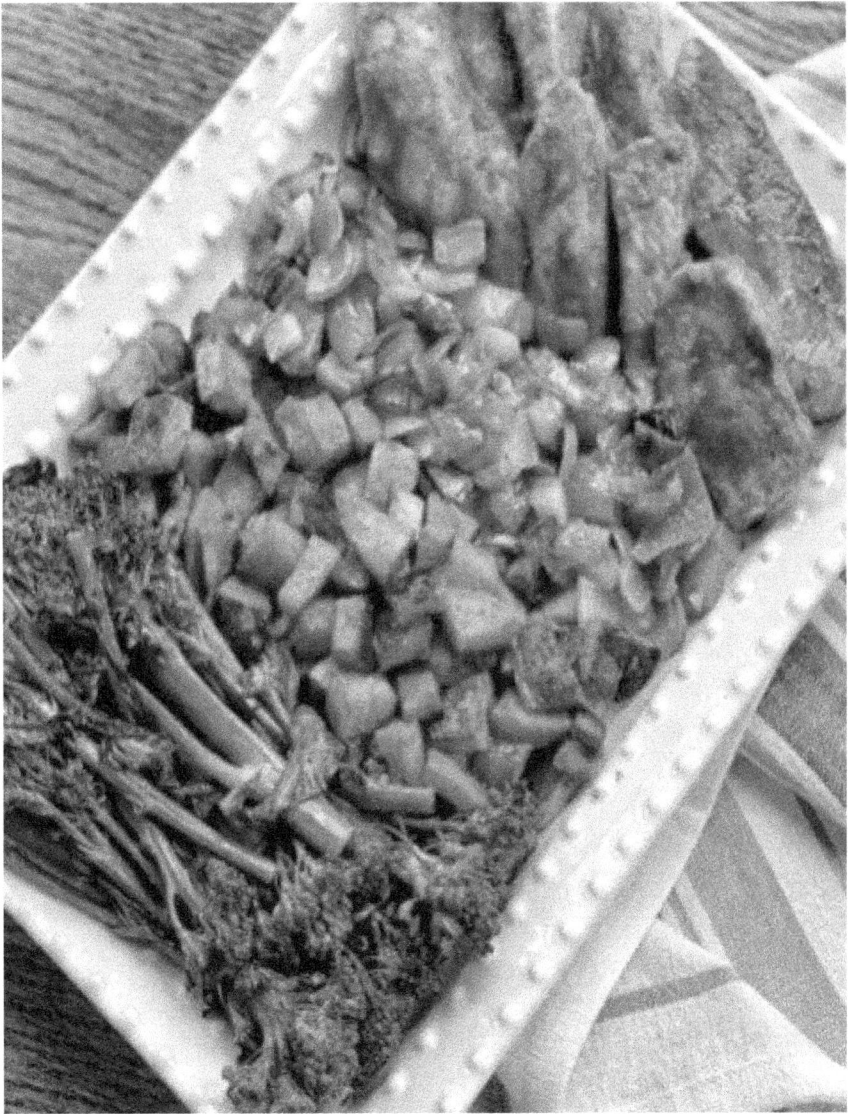

Chapter 2

Your 30-Day Weight Loss Meal Plan (How It's Structured)

Most meal plans fail for one simple reason: they demand too many decisions. Too many choices create fatigue, and fatigue leads to inconsistency. This 30-day plan is built to remove that burden. It is not designed to impress—it is designed to be followed.

Everything here is intentional. The structure exists so you can focus on eating, not overthinking.

How the 30 Days Are Organized for Ease

The plan is divided into four simple weeks. Each week follows a familiar rhythm: breakfast, lunch, and dinner are clearly defined, using the same core ingredients in different combinations.

You are not expected to reinvent your meals daily. Instead, the plan:

- Uses a small group of proteins repeatedly
- Rotates vegetables to keep meals fresh
- Keeps cooking methods simple and predictable

Each day builds on the previous one. By the second week, meals feel familiar. By the third week, they feel automatic. That sense of ease is not accidental—it is the foundation of success.

Why Meals Repeat Strategically (Less Thinking, Better Adherence)

Repetition is not laziness. It is strategy.

When meals repeat:

- Grocery shopping becomes faster

- Cooking time drops significantly

- Decision fatigue disappears

- Consistency improves naturally

Weight loss does not require constant novelty. It requires reliable habits. Repeating meals allows your body to settle into a rhythm and your mind to relax around food.

You will notice that the same breakfasts or lunches may appear multiple times a week. This is deliberate. Familiar meals reduce stress and increase follow-through.

How to Swap Meals Without Breaking the Plan

Life happens. Schedules change. Ingredients run out. The plan accounts for that.

You can safely swap meals as long as you follow one rule:

keep the structure the same.

For example:

- Breakfast stays protein-focused

- Lunch stays balanced and filling

- Dinner remains simple and protein-forward

If you swap chicken for fish, eggs for yogurt, or beef for turkey, you are still aligned. The plan is flexible within its framework. One missed meal does not undo progress— returning to structure does.

Eating Out or Busy-Day Adjustments

There will be days when cooking isn't realistic. The goal is not perfection—it is alignment.

On busy days:

- Choose grilled or roasted protein

- Add vegetables if available

- Skip sugary drinks and refined sides

Restaurants, takeout, and social meals do not ruin progress when approached calmly. Make the best available choice, eat until satisfied, and move on without guilt.

This plan does not punish real life—it works with it.

What to Drink During the Plan

Hydration supports appetite control and energy, but it does not need to be complicated.

Stick to:

- Water
- Sparkling water
- Unsweetened tea
- Black coffee (if tolerated)

Avoid:

- Sugary drinks

- Juice

- Sweetened beverages disguised as "healthy"

Drinks should support meals, not replace them or quietly add calories.

Why This Structure Works

This plan succeeds because it respects reality. It removes guesswork, simplifies decisions, and allows repetition to do the heavy lifting.

You are not starting a diet—you are following a system.

And systems are easier to maintain than motivation.

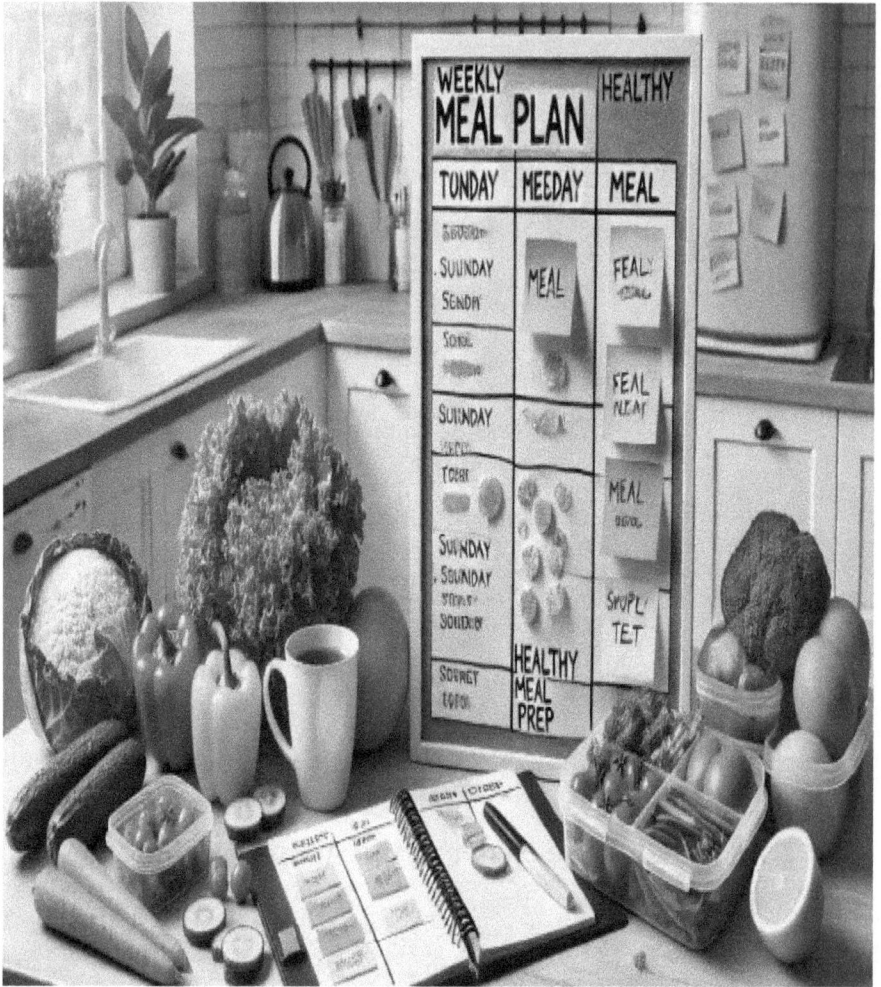

PART I: BREAKFASTS THAT KEEP YOU FULL

Chapter 3

High-Protein Breakfasts (Days 1–30)

Breakfast sets the tone for the entire day. When the first meal is rushed, sugar-heavy, or built without protein, hunger shows up early—and it shows up loud. Cravings creep in. Energy dips. Decisions get harder as the day goes on.

This chapter exists to prevent that chain reaction.

High-protein breakfasts don't need to be complicated, expensive, or time-consuming. They need to be reliable. When protein anchors your morning, appetite settles, energy steadies, and the rest of the day becomes easier to manage.

Why Breakfast Protein Matters for Appetite Control

Protein has a unique effect on hunger hormones. It slows digestion, keeps you full longer, and reduces the urge to snack between meals. Starting your day with adequate protein is one of the simplest ways to reduce overall calorie intake—without trying to eat less.

This isn't about forcing breakfast if you're not hungry. It's about making breakfast work for you when you do eat it.

When protein is present in the morning:

- Cravings are quieter
- Energy lasts longer
- Lunch decisions improve automatically

That's leverage—and leverage makes consistency easier.

Simple Morning Meals Ready in 5–15 Minutes

Mornings don't allow for complexity. These breakfasts are

designed to fit real schedules.

Most recipes in this chapter:

- Use a small number of ingredients
- Cook quickly on the stovetop or require no cooking at all
- Can be repeated several times a week without boredom

You'll find meals you can prepare fresh in minutes, along with options you can assemble the night before and grab on the way out.

No Powders Required (Protein Comes from Food)

This plan does not rely on protein powders, shakes, or bars. Protein comes from food you recognize and trust—eggs, dairy, and whole ingredients you can buy at any local grocery store.

This matters because food-based protein:

- Is more satisfying

- Encourages normal eating habits

- Feels sustainable long-term

If you ever choose to include supplements later, that's a personal choice. But nothing in this book depends on them.

Recipe Types Included

This chapter rotates a small group of dependable breakfast styles so mornings stay easy without feeling repetitive.

Egg-Based Breakfasts

Simple scrambles, pan-fried eggs, and baked egg dishes form the backbone of many mornings. Eggs are affordable, versatile, and naturally rich in protein.

Greek Yogurt Bowls

Greek yogurt provides a thick, filling base that pairs well with nuts, seeds, and fruit. These bowls are fast, cooling, and especially useful on busy mornings.

Cottage Cheese Plates

Cottage cheese is an underrated protein powerhouse. Paired with vegetables or healthy fats, it creates a surprisingly satisfying breakfast.

Simple Breakfast Scrambles

Quick skillet meals using eggs and vegetables—perfect for using leftovers and reducing food waste.

Make-Ahead Options for Busy

Mornings

Egg muffins and pre-prepped components allow you to eat well even when time is tight.

30-Day Breakfast Rotation (Examples)

The breakfasts repeat strategically across the 30 days to reduce decision fatigue while keeping meals enjoyable.

You'll see options like:

- Scrambled eggs with spinach and feta
- Greek yogurt with nuts and berries
- Cottage cheese with sliced avocado and tomatoes
- Egg muffins with mixed vegetables
- Pan-fried eggs with sautéed mushrooms

These meals rotate naturally. You don't need a different breakfast every day—you need a few good ones you can rely on.

Every ingredient listed is widely available, affordable, and familiar. No specialty shopping required.

How to Use This Chapter

Pick a few favorites. Repeat them. Keep it simple.

If mornings are hectic, lean on make-ahead options. If you enjoy cooking, rotate through fresh scrambles. Either way, the goal is the same: start the day full, steady, and confident.

Once breakfast stops being a problem, the rest of the plan becomes easier to follow.

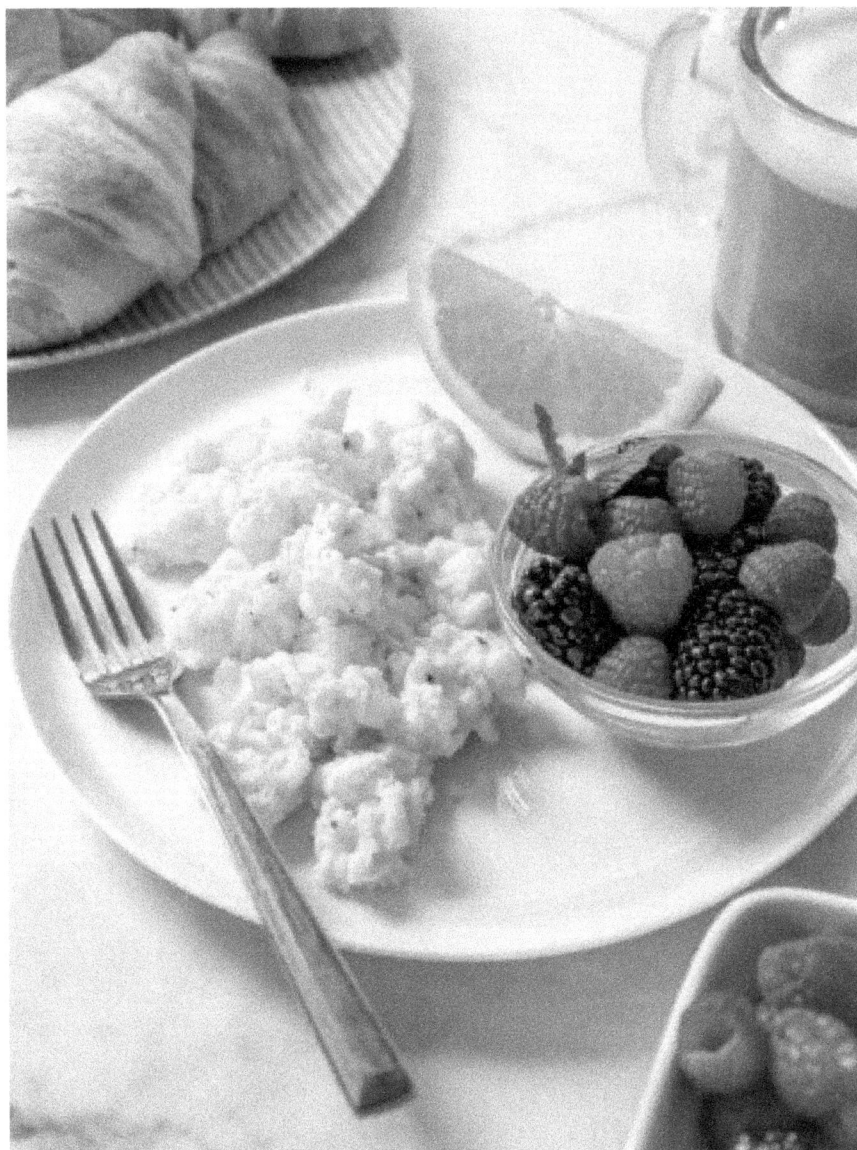

PART II: SATISFYING LUNCHES THAT

PREVENT SNACKING

Chapter 4

Protein-Focused Lunches for Steady Energy

Lunch is where many weight-loss plans quietly fall apart. Not because people overeat—but because meals are built around convenience instead of nourishment. A bread-heavy lunch may feel quick and harmless, yet it often leads to a mid-afternoon crash, creeping hunger, and unnecessary snacking before dinner.

This chapter resets that pattern.

Protein-focused lunches provide steady energy, stable appetite, and mental clarity for the rest of the day. They are filling without being heavy, practical without being boring, and designed to work whether you're at home, at work, or on the move.

How to Build a Filling Lunch Without Bread Overload

Bread is often used as the structure of lunch—sandwiches, wraps, rolls. In this plan, **protein becomes the structure instead.**

A filling lunch follows one clear principle:

Protein first, vegetables second, extras last.

When protein anchors the meal:

- Hunger stays controlled for hours
- Energy remains steady
- Afternoon cravings fade naturally

Vegetables add volume and fiber. Healthy fats add satisfaction. Bread is not forbidden—but it is no longer the centerpiece. Once protein takes the lead, lunches stop feeling light but unsatisfying.

Packable Lunches for Work or Home

Lunch should travel well. These meals are designed to hold up in containers, reheat easily, or taste just as good cold.

Most lunches in this chapter:

- Can be prepared ahead

- Require minimal assembly

- Use ingredients that overlap with dinner recipes

This means fewer groceries, less cooking time, and more consistency. Whether you're packing lunch for work or grabbing something from the fridge at home, the structure remains the same.

Leftover-Friendly Meals

Cooking once and eating twice is not a shortcut—it's a strategy.

Many lunches are intentionally built from dinner leftovers:

- Grilled chicken becomes tomorrow's bowl

- Roasted vegetables turn into a warm skillet

- Cooked protein pairs easily with fresh elements

This approach saves time and keeps meals aligned without additional effort. When leftovers are planned, lunch becomes automatic.

Recipe Types Included

This chapter offers a small set of dependable lunch styles that repeat comfortably across the 30 days.

Chicken Bowls

Simple, balanced, and endlessly adaptable. Chicken pairs easily with vegetables and light sauces for filling meals that don't weigh you down.

Tuna and Salmon Plates

These meals are fast, protein-dense, and require minimal cooking. Perfect for days when time is limited but energy matters.

Turkey and Veggie Skillets

Warm, comforting lunches that feel substantial without excess carbs. Ideal for cooler days or when you want something hearty.

Simple Salads with Real Protein

These are not side salads. Protein takes center stage, supported by vegetables and healthy fats to keep you full.

Warm Lunch Options for Comfort

Not every lunch needs to be cold. Warm meals can increase satisfaction and reduce the urge to snack later.

30-Day Lunch Rotation (Examples)

Lunches rotate deliberately across the month to reduce decision fatigue while keeping flavors familiar.

You'll see meals such as:

- Grilled chicken with mixed vegetables
- Tuna salad with olive oil and lemon
- Turkey and zucchini skillet
- Salmon with cucumber and yogurt sauce
- Egg and avocado protein bowls

These meals are simple, recognizable, and easy to repeat. Ingredients are widely available at local grocery stores, making the plan accessible and affordable.

How to Use This Chapter

Choose a few lunches you enjoy. Repeat them confidently. Let leftovers do the work when possible.

When lunch is steady and satisfying, the rest of the day becomes easier. Energy stays level. Cravings stay quiet. And dinner decisions feel calmer.

That's not discipline—that's good structure.

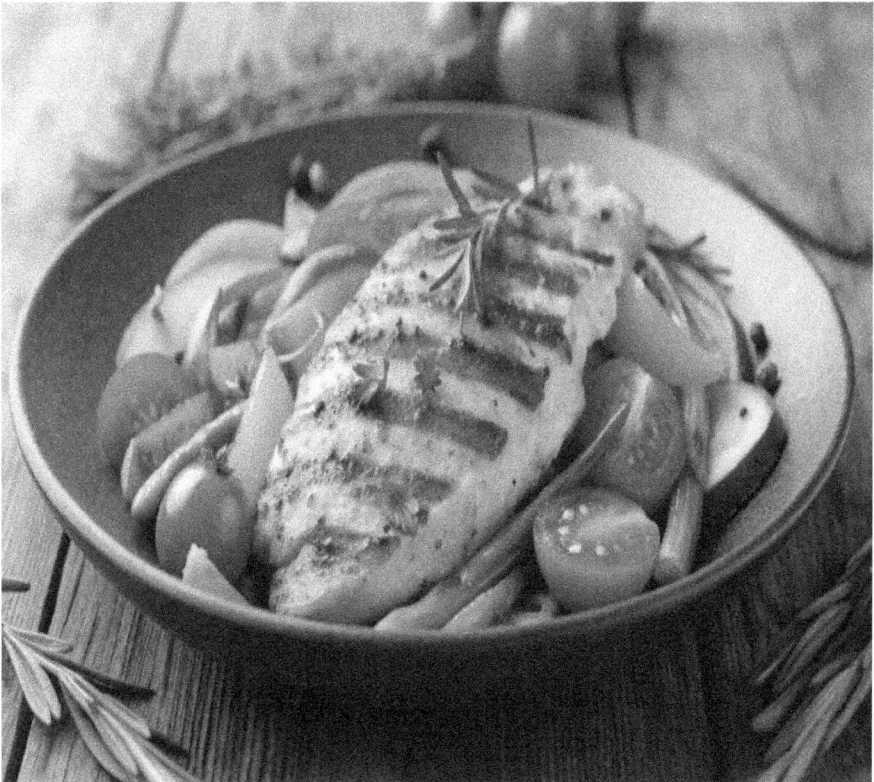

PART III: SIMPLE DINNERS THAT SUPPORT FAT LOSS

Chapter 5

Easy High-Protein Dinners (No Fancy Cooking)

Dinner is where many people expect weight loss to feel hardest. Long days create big appetites, comfort cravings, and a desire for something filling and familiar. Too often, that leads to meals that are heavy, oversized, or built around convenience foods that undo the day's progress.

This chapter takes a different approach.

Dinner does not need to be complicated—or restrictive—to be satisfying. When protein leads and cooking stays simple, evening meals become grounding instead of guilt-driven. You eat well, feel full, and still move closer to your goals.

Why Dinner Doesn't Need to Be Heavy to Be

Satisfying

Satisfaction doesn't come from eating the most food—it comes from eating the right structure.

A protein-forward dinner:

- Signals fullness sooner

- Prevents late-night snacking

- Supports recovery and muscle maintenance

- Feels comforting without being overwhelming

When meals are balanced and calm, you finish dinner satisfied instead of stuffed. That feeling matters. It builds trust with food and makes consistency easier the next day.

One-Pan and Stovetop Meals

Dinner should not feel like a project.

Most recipes in this chapter are designed to:

- Use one pan or one baking tray

- Cook on the stovetop or in the oven
- Require minimal prep and cleanup

Simple cooking methods reduce friction. Less mess means less resistance—and less resistance means you're more likely to cook at home consistently.

Comfort-Style Dishes Made Lighter

Comfort food doesn't need to disappear. It just needs to be adjusted.

These dinners keep familiar flavors while shifting the balance:

- Protein becomes the main focus
- Vegetables add volume and texture
- Refined carbs are reduced or removed

You still get warmth, satisfaction, and familiarity—without the heaviness that lingers into the evening.

Recipe Types Included

This chapter rotates dependable dinner styles that work across busy weekdays and slower evenings.

Baked Chicken and Fish

Oven-baked meals are reliable, hands-off, and easy to repeat. Season, bake, and let the oven do the work.

Beef and Vegetable Skillets

One-pan meals that feel hearty and grounding. Protein-rich, filling, and ideal for nights when you want something substantial.

Simple Stir-Fries

Quick-cooking meals that use fresh vegetables and lean

protein. Flavorful without being complicated.

Sheet-Pan Meals

Protein and vegetables cooked together for maximum convenience and minimal cleanup.

Slow Evenings, Minimal Cleanup

These dinners respect your energy level at the end of the day. You shouldn't need motivation to cook—just a simple plan.

30-Day Dinner Rotation (Examples)

Dinner options rotate throughout the month to keep meals familiar and manageable.

You'll see meals like:

- Baked chicken thighs with roasted vegetables

- Pan-seared fish with garlic greens

- Ground beef and cabbage skillet

- Chicken stir-fry with peppers

- Turkey meatballs with zucchini

These recipes rely on basic techniques and widely available ingredients. Nothing exotic. Nothing intimidating. Just solid dinners you can cook again and again.

How to Use This Chapter

Dinner does not need variety every night—it needs reliability.

Pick a few dinners you enjoy. Rotate them. Repeat them. Let simplicity work in your favor.

When evenings feel calm and satisfying, weight loss stops feeling like a battle—and starts feeling sustainable.

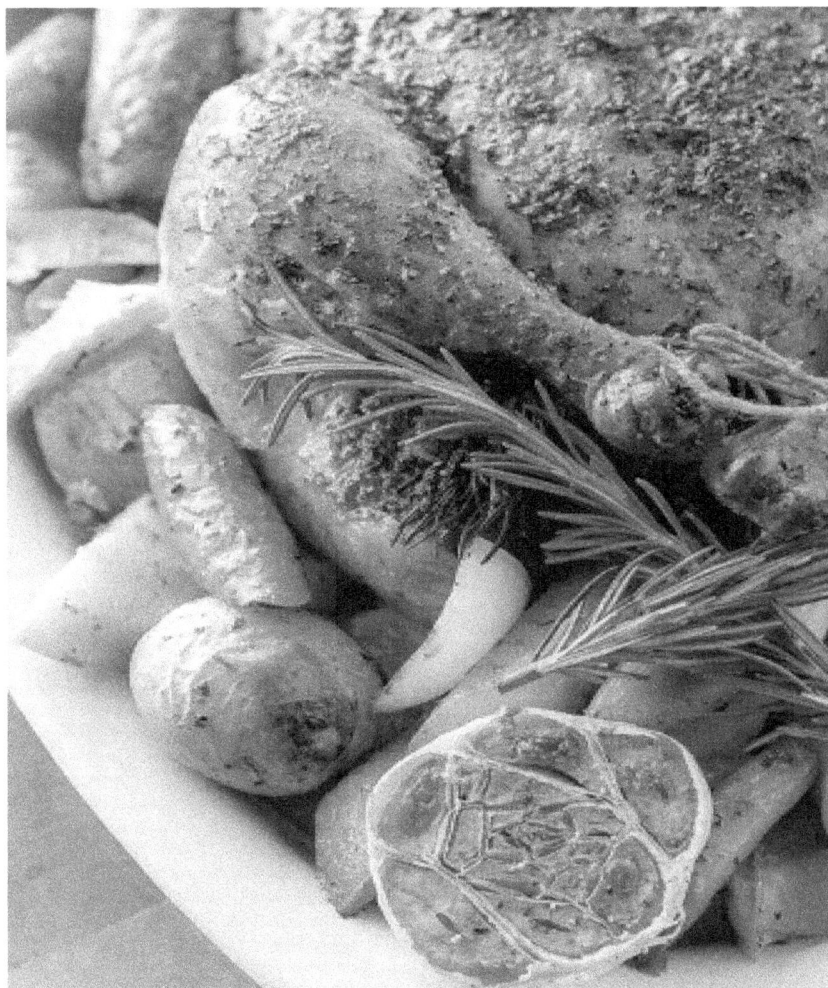

PART IV: WEEK-BY-WEEK 30-DAY MEAL PLAN

Chapter 6

Week 1 – Reset and Simplicity

The first week is not about perfection. It is about settling in. Your body is adjusting, your appetite cues are recalibrating, and your mind is learning that meals can be satisfying without excess. Simplicity is the goal—because simplicity is what you can repeat.

This week uses familiar foods, gentle repetition, and straightforward cooking to remove friction and build momentum.

Your Full 7-Day Plan (Breakfast, Lunch, Dinner)

Below is a clear, no-guesswork outline for the first seven days. Meals repeat intentionally to make shopping and cooking easier.

Day 1

- **Breakfast:** Scrambled eggs with spinach
- **Lunch:** Grilled chicken with mixed vegetables
- **Dinner:** Baked chicken thighs with roasted vegetables

Day 2

- **Breakfast:** Greek yogurt with nuts and berries
- **Lunch:** Tuna salad with olive oil and lemon
- **Dinner:** Ground beef and cabbage skillet

Day 3

- **Breakfast:** Cottage cheese with avocado and tomatoes
- **Lunch:** Turkey and zucchini skillet
- **Dinner:** Pan-seared fish with garlic greens

Day 4

- **Breakfast:** Egg muffins with vegetables

- **Lunch:** Egg and avocado protein bowl

- **Dinner:** Chicken stir-fry with peppers

Day 5

- **Breakfast:** Scrambled eggs with mushrooms

- **Lunch:** Grilled chicken leftovers with vegetables

- **Dinner:** Turkey meatballs with zucchini

Day 6

- **Breakfast:** Greek yogurt with seeds

- **Lunch:** Salmon with cucumber and yogurt sauce

- **Dinner:** Sheet-pan chicken and vegetables

Day 7

- **Breakfast:** Pan-fried eggs with sautéed greens

- **Lunch:** Tuna or chicken salad

- **Dinner:** Simple beef and vegetable skillet

Meals are interchangeable within the same category if

needed. Keep the structure—protein first—and you remain aligned.

Grocery List Guidance (Shop Once, Eat All Week)

Week 1 is designed so you can shop once and reuse ingredients across multiple meals.

Proteins

- Eggs
- Chicken thighs or breasts
- Ground beef
- Turkey
- Fish (salmon or white fish)
- Greek yogurt
- Cottage cheese
- Canned tuna

Vegetables

- Spinach or leafy greens

- Zucchini

- Bell peppers

- Mushrooms

- Cabbage

- Mixed vegetables (fresh or frozen)

Fats & Basics

- Olive oil

- Simple spices (salt, pepper, garlic, herbs)

This short list keeps the kitchen stocked without overwhelm and reduces food waste.

What to Expect in the First Week (Hunger, Energy, Adjustments)

The first few days may feel different—and that's normal.

You may notice:

- Hunger patterns shifting

- Cravings for refined carbs fading gradually
- Energy stabilizing instead of spiking and crashing

Some people feel lighter quickly. Others feel fuller sooner. Both are normal responses. The key is not reacting emotionally to early sensations. Your body is learning a new rhythm.

Eat when hungry. Stop when satisfied. Drink water regularly. Trust the structure.

By the end of Week 1, meals will feel less uncertain—and that calm is the first real sign of progress.

How to Approach This Week

Keep it simple. Don't add extras. Don't chase variety.

The goal is not excitement—it's **ease.**

When the first week feels manageable, the rest of the plan becomes easier to follow.

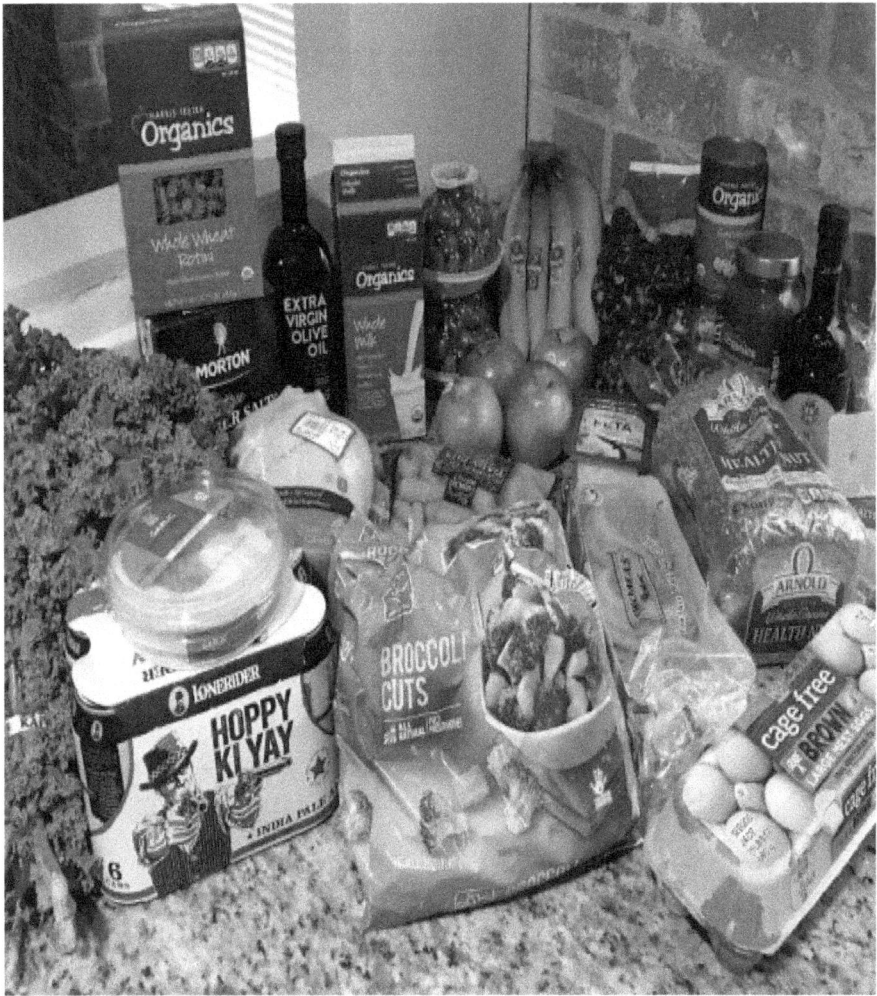

Chapter 7

Week 2 – Consistency Builds Momentum

By the time you reach Week 2, something important has shifted. Meals no longer feel unfamiliar. You're not wondering what to eat or whether you're doing it "right." The structure is starting to work quietly in the background—and that's exactly the point.

This week is about **reinforcement.** Not tightening rules. Not adding complexity. Just repeating what works until it becomes natural.

Momentum is built through consistency, not effort.

Your Full 7-Day Plan (Week 2)

Week 2 continues the same reliable framework from Week 1, with slight rotations to keep meals enjoyable while maintaining ease.

Day 8

- **Breakfast:** Scrambled eggs with spinach and feta
- **Lunch:** Grilled chicken with mixed vegetables
- **Dinner:** Pan-seared fish with garlic greens

Day 9

- **Breakfast:** Greek yogurt with nuts and berries
- **Lunch:** Tuna salad with olive oil and lemon
- **Dinner:** Ground beef and cabbage skillet

Day 10

- **Breakfast:** Cottage cheese with avocado and tomatoes
- **Lunch:** Turkey and zucchini skillet
- **Dinner:** Baked chicken thighs with roasted vegetables

Day 11

- **Breakfast:** Egg muffins with vegetables

- **Lunch:** Egg and avocado protein bowl

- **Dinner:** Chicken stir-fry with peppers

Day 12

- **Breakfast:** Scrambled eggs with mushrooms

- **Lunch:** Salmon with cucumber and yogurt sauce

- **Dinner:** Turkey meatballs with zucchini

Day 13

- **Breakfast:** Greek yogurt with seeds

- **Lunch:** Chicken leftovers with vegetables

- **Dinner:** Sheet-pan chicken and vegetables

Day 14

- **Breakfast:** Pan-fried eggs with sautéed greens

- **Lunch:** Tuna or chicken salad

- **Dinner:** Simple beef and vegetable skillet

Meals can be swapped within categories if needed. Keep

the protein-first structure, and the plan stays intact.

Why Repeating Meals Works (And Why It Matters Now)

By Week 2, repetition becomes an advantage instead of a limitation.

- Repeating meals:
- Reduces decision fatigue
- Makes grocery shopping faster
- Improves portion awareness naturally
- Helps appetite cues settle

Your body thrives on predictability. When meals are consistent, hunger becomes more reliable—and that reliability is what prevents overeating.

You are no longer relying on motivation. You are relying on routine.

Staying Full Without Snacking

One of the quiet wins of Week 2 is realizing that snacking becomes less necessary.

When meals are built correctly:

- Protein keeps you full longer

- Balanced fats slow digestion

- Vegetables add volume without heaviness

If hunger shows up between meals, pause before reacting. Ask whether it's true hunger or habit. Often, a glass of water or a short break is enough.

If you are genuinely hungry, eat your next meal without guilt. This plan is not about resisting hunger—it's about **preventing it**.

What You May Notice This Week

Many people experience:

- Fewer cravings

- More stable energy

- A calmer relationship with food

- Less mental noise around eating

Weight loss may or may not feel dramatic yet—and that's okay. What matters is that the process feels manageable. Sustainable progress often feels almost uneventful.

That's a good sign.

How to Approach Week 2

Trust the repetition. Don't chase novelty. Let the structure carry you.

When eating becomes routine, consistency becomes effortless—and momentum takes care of itself.

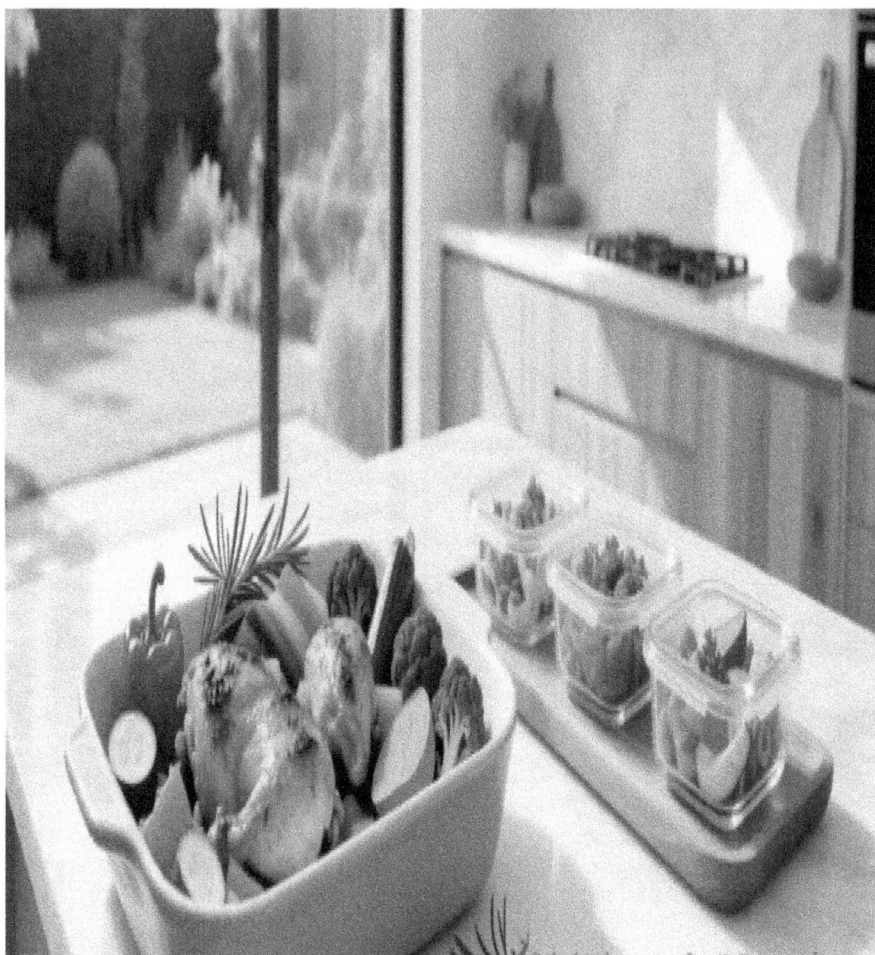

Chapter 8

Week 3 – Confidence and Rhythm

Week 3 is where confidence quietly replaces effort. By now, meals feel familiar. You're no longer second-guessing portions or wondering whether you're doing things "right." The plan has a rhythm—and your body has started to trust it.

This is the week where eating well stops feeling like a project and starts feeling normal.

Your Full 7-Day Plan (Week 3)

Week 3 continues the same dependable structure, with gentle rotation to maintain ease and enjoyment.

Day 15

- **Breakfast:** Scrambled eggs with spinach

- **Lunch:** Grilled chicken with mixed vegetables
- **Dinner:** Baked chicken thighs with roasted vegetables

Day 16

- **Breakfast:** Greek yogurt with nuts and berries
- **Lunch:** Tuna salad with olive oil and lemon
- **Dinner:** Pan-seared fish with garlic greens

Day 17

- **Breakfast:** Cottage cheese with avocado and tomatoes
- **Lunch:** Turkey and zucchini skillet
- **Dinner:** Ground beef and cabbage skillet

Day 18

- **Breakfast:** Egg muffins with vegetables
- **Lunch:** Egg and avocado protein bowl
- **Dinner:** Chicken stir-fry with peppers

Day 19

- **Breakfast:** Scrambled eggs with mushrooms
- **Lunch:** Salmon with cucumber and yogurt sauce
- **Dinner:** Turkey meatballs with zucchini

Day 20

- **Breakfast:** Greek yogurt with seeds
- **Lunch:** Chicken leftovers with vegetables
- **Dinner:** Sheet-pan chicken and vegetables

Day 21

- **Breakfast:** Pan-fried eggs with sautéed greens
- **Lunch:** Tuna or chicken salad
- **Dinner:** Simple beef and vegetable skillet

Meals can be swapped within the same category when needed. The structure—not perfection—is what keeps progress steady.

How Appetite Naturally Stabilizes

One of the most noticeable changes in Week 3 is how hunger feels different.

You may notice:

- Fewer intense cravings

- Hunger arriving more predictably

- Feeling satisfied with simpler meals

- Less urge to snack between meals

This happens because protein-forward meals and consistent timing allow hunger signals to regulate themselves. You're no longer riding blood sugar highs and crashes. Appetite becomes calmer—and easier to trust.

At this stage, many people realize they are eating less without trying to. That's not restraint. That's alignment.

Eating Out Adjustments (If Needed)

By Week 3, you've learned the structure well enough to apply it anywhere.

When eating out:

- Choose grilled, baked, or pan-seared protein
- Add vegetables if available
- Skip sugary drinks and heavy sauces when possible

You don't need to find the "perfect" option. Make the best available choice, eat until comfortably full, and move on. One meal does not undo weeks of consistency.

This confidence matters. It's what allows the plan to work in real life—not just at home.

What This Week Represents

Week 3 isn't about pushing harder. It's about recognizing that the system is working.

Food feels simpler. Choices feel clearer. And weight loss, when it happens, feels like a side effect—not a struggle.

That sense of rhythm is what makes progress sustainable.

How to Approach Week 3

Stay the course. Don't change what's working.

Confidence doesn't come from control—it comes from repetition. And by now, repetition has done its job.

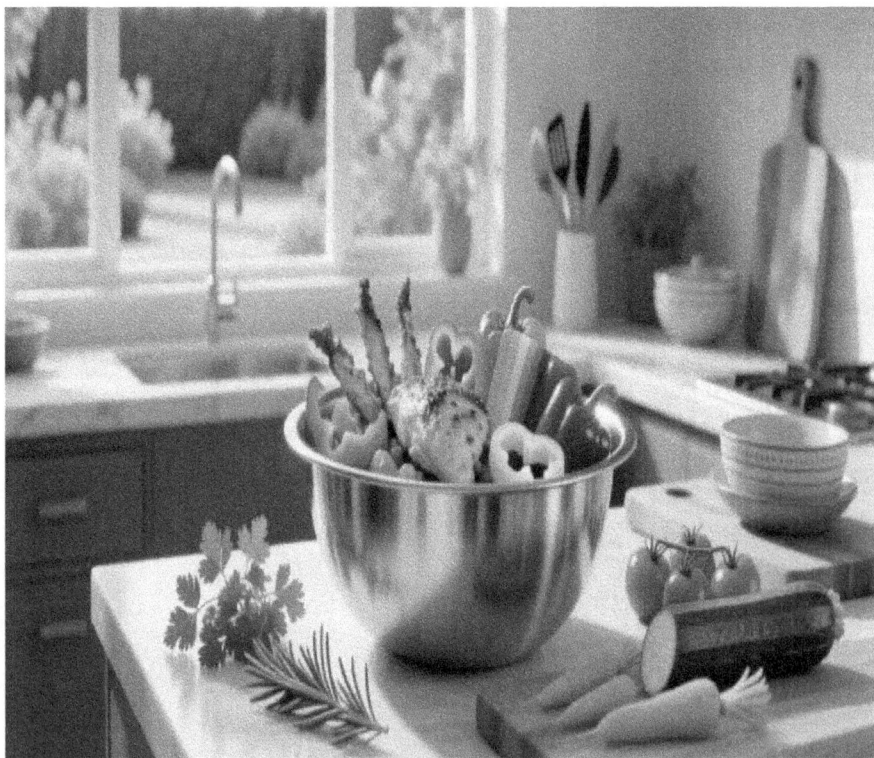

Chapter 9

Week 4 – Making It Sustainable

Week 4 is not about pushing harder—it's about settling in. By now, eating this way no longer feels like a temporary plan. It feels workable. Familiar. Calm. That's the signal you've been building toward.

This final week is about continuity. The goal is not to "finish" the plan, but to step out of it with habits you can carry forward without friction.

Your Final 7-Day Plan (Week 4)

The structure remains steady. Meals repeat because repetition is what makes progress sustainable—not novelty.

Day 22

- **Breakfast:** Scrambled eggs with spinach and feta

- **Lunch:** Grilled chicken with mixed vegetables

- **Dinner:** Pan-seared fish with garlic greens

Day 23

- **Breakfast:** Greek yogurt with nuts and berries

- **Lunch:** Tuna salad with olive oil and lemon

- **Dinner:** Ground beef and cabbage skillet

Day 24

- **Breakfast:** Cottage cheese with avocado and tomatoes

- **Lunch:** Turkey and zucchini skillet

- **Dinner:** Baked chicken thighs with roasted vegetables

Day 25

- **Breakfast:** Egg muffins with vegetables

- **Lunch:** Egg and avocado protein bowl

- **Dinner:** Chicken stir-fry with peppers

Day 26

- **Breakfast:** Scrambled eggs with mushrooms

- **Lunch:** Salmon with cucumber and yogurt sauce

- **Dinner:** Turkey meatballs with zucchini

Day 27

- **Breakfast:** Greek yogurt with seeds

- **Lunch:** Chicken leftovers with vegetables

- **Dinner:** Sheet-pan chicken and vegetables

Day 28

- **Breakfast:** Pan-fried eggs with sautéed greens

- **Lunch:** Tuna or chicken salad

- **Dinner:** Simple beef and vegetable skillet

Use swaps if needed. Keep the protein-first structure. Consistency matters more than precision.

How to Continue Beyond Day 30

The end of the 30 days is not a stopping point—it's a checkpoint.

You now have:

- Reliable breakfast options

- Dependable lunches that keep energy steady

- Simple dinners you can cook without stress

To continue:

- Repeat the 30-day cycle

- Mix and match favorite meals

- Maintain the same structure with new ingredients if desired

There is no requirement to "move on" to something else. If a system works, you keep using it.

Transitioning Into Long-Term Habits

Sustainability comes from a few core habits—not rigid rules.

Carry these forward:

- Build meals around protein
- Keep refined carbs occasional, not automatic
- Eat until satisfied, not stuffed
- Shop simply and cook repeatedly

Some days will be more flexible than others. That's normal. Progress is maintained by returning to structure—not by avoiding deviation entirely.

The difference now is confidence. You know how to eat in a way that supports your body without drama.

What Success Really Looks Like

By Week 4, success isn't just about the scale.

It looks like:

- Less mental noise around food
- Fewer cravings
- More stable energy
- Meals that feel easy instead of effortful

That ease is the real win. When eating well no longer requires motivation, results become durable.

How to Move Forward

There is no "after" this plan—only continuation.

Repeat what works. Adjust when life demands it. Return to simplicity when things drift.

That's how weight loss becomes sustainable—not through intensity, but through calm consistency.

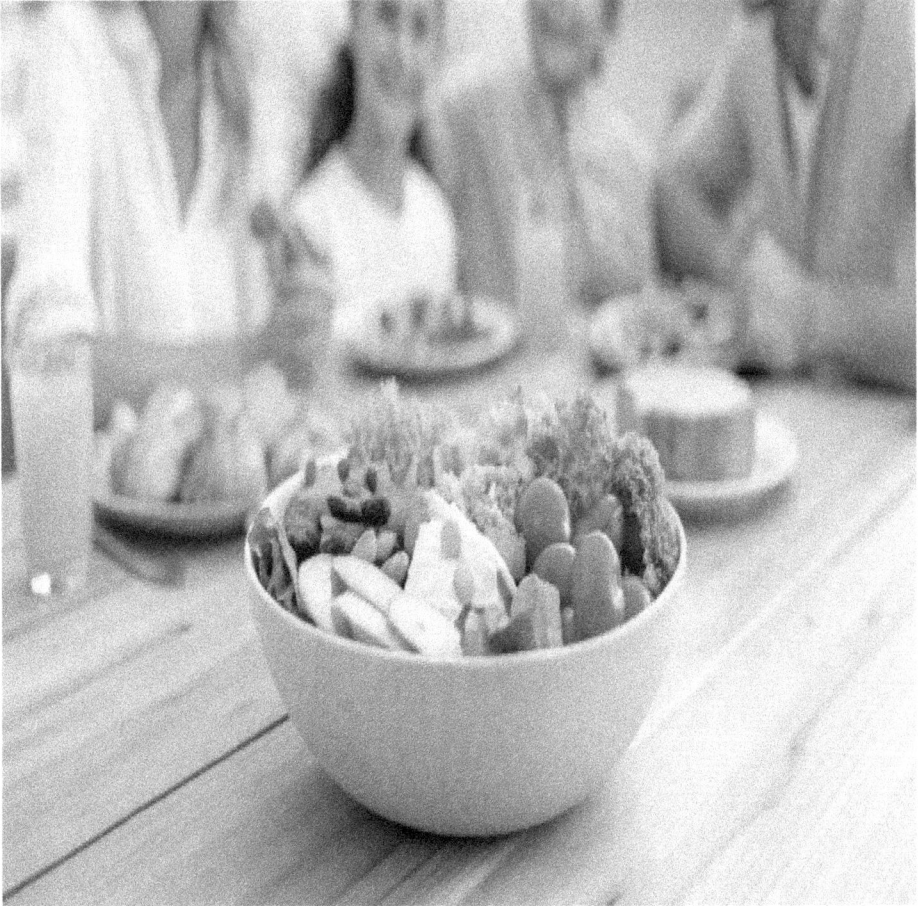

Chapter 10

After the 30 Days – How to Keep the Weight Off

The most important question isn't whether the 30 days worked.

It's **what happens next.**

Many people lose weight only to gain it back because the plan ends—and nothing replaces it. This chapter exists to prevent that cycle. The goal now is not continued restriction, but **continuity**. You're no longer "on" a plan. You're living with a structure that supports your weight naturally.

How to Repeat the Plan (Without Burnout)

If the past 30 days felt manageable—and for most people, they do—the simplest option is to repeat them.

Repeating the plan works because:

- Meals are already familiar
- Grocery shopping is efficient
- Cooking feels automatic
- Appetite is already regulated

You can repeat the full 30 days exactly as written, or rotate only your favorite breakfasts, lunches, and dinners. There is no requirement to change what is working. Progress doesn't demand novelty—it demands reliability.

Some people repeat the plan continuously. Others repeat it during the week and loosen structure slightly on weekends. Both approaches work when protein remains the anchor.

When and How to Add Carbs Back Carefully

Carbs don't need to be avoided forever—but they do need to be reintroduced intentionally.

The right time to add carbs back is when:

- Hunger feels stable

- Cravings are quiet

- Portions feel natural

Start small and strategic:

- Add one carb source to one meal per day

- Choose whole-food carbs over refined ones

- Observe how your appetite responds

Good reintroduction options include:

- Beans or lentils

- Sweet potatoes

- Whole grains in modest portions

If hunger spikes or cravings return, simply scale back and return to the previous structure. There is no failure in adjusting—only feedback.

Protein Habits for Long-Term Success

Protein remains the foundation beyond weight loss.

Long-term success comes from:

Including protein at every meal

Prioritizing whole-food sources

Letting protein guide portion sizes naturally

Protein stabilizes appetite, supports muscle, and prevents the slow creep of overeating that leads to rebound weight gain. When protein stays consistent, flexibility becomes safer.

This is why protein-first eating is not a phase—it's a lifestyle anchor.

Avoiding Rebound Weight Gain

Rebound weight gain doesn't happen overnight. It happens quietly when structure disappears.

To avoid it:

- Keep meal timing predictable
- Maintain a few go-to meals you repeat often
- Notice hunger changes early
- Return to simplicity when weight or appetite drifts

You don't need to correct everything at once. One protein-focused day can reset momentum quickly. Small corrections are far more effective than extreme reactions.

What Maintenance Really Means

Maintenance is not holding your breath at a certain number.

It's:

- Eating in a way that feels calm
- Adjusting without panic
- Returning to structure without guilt

The reason this plan works long-term is because it doesn't rely on motivation. It relies on habits that feel reasonable even when life gets busy.

Moving Forward With Confidence

You now know how to eat without guesswork.

If weight changes, you know how to respond.

If life interrupts structure, you know how to return.

If hunger shifts, you know what to anchor to.

That knowledge is what keeps weight off—not discipline, not restriction, and not fear.

Bonus Section

Simple Swaps & Emergency Meals

Life doesn't pause for meal plans. Ingredients run out. Schedules change. Stress spikes. This bonus section exists for those moments—not to "save" the plan, but to keep it intact without effort.

You don't need perfect conditions to stay consistent. You need options that work when things go sideways.

Fast Protein Swaps When Ingredients Are Missing

When a planned protein isn't available, the solution is not to skip the meal or grab something random. It's to **swap within the same role**.

Think in categories, not recipes.

If you're missing:

- **Chicken** → use eggs, tuna, turkey, or yogurt

- **Fish** → use eggs, cottage cheese, or ground meat

- **Fresh meat** → use canned protein or leftovers

- **Cooked protein** → use dairy-based protein temporarily

As long as protein remains the anchor of the meal, the structure holds. Vegetables and fats adjust naturally around it.

No recalculating. No starting over.

10-Minute Emergency Meals

These meals exist for busy evenings, late afternoons, or days when energy is low but hunger is real.

Examples of reliable emergency meals:

- Scrambled eggs with frozen vegetables

- Greek yogurt with nuts and seeds

- Tuna mixed with olive oil and vegetables

- Cottage cheese with avocado and tomatoes
- Leftover protein reheated with vegetables

They aren't fancy. They aren't impressive. They **are effective**.

Emergency meals prevent the spiral that starts with "I'll just grab something quick" and ends with regret. Eating something simple and protein-focused is always better than skipping or overcomplicating.

What to Do on High-Stress Days

Stress changes appetite. Sometimes it increases hunger. Sometimes it kills it. Both responses are normal.

On high-stress days:

- Stick to familiar meals
- Avoid experimenting with new foods
- Eat earlier if hunger shows up sooner
- Keep portions steady, not reactive

This is not the time to push harder or restrict more. Stress is already taxing your system. The goal is stability, not control.

If all you do on a stressful day is eat three simple protein-based meals, that is success.

The Real Purpose of This Section

This section exists to remove fear.

Fear of missing ingredients.

Fear of busy days.

Fear of stress undoing progress.

When you know how to adjust calmly, consistency becomes durable. You stop reacting emotionally—and start responding practically.

That's how weight loss survives real life.

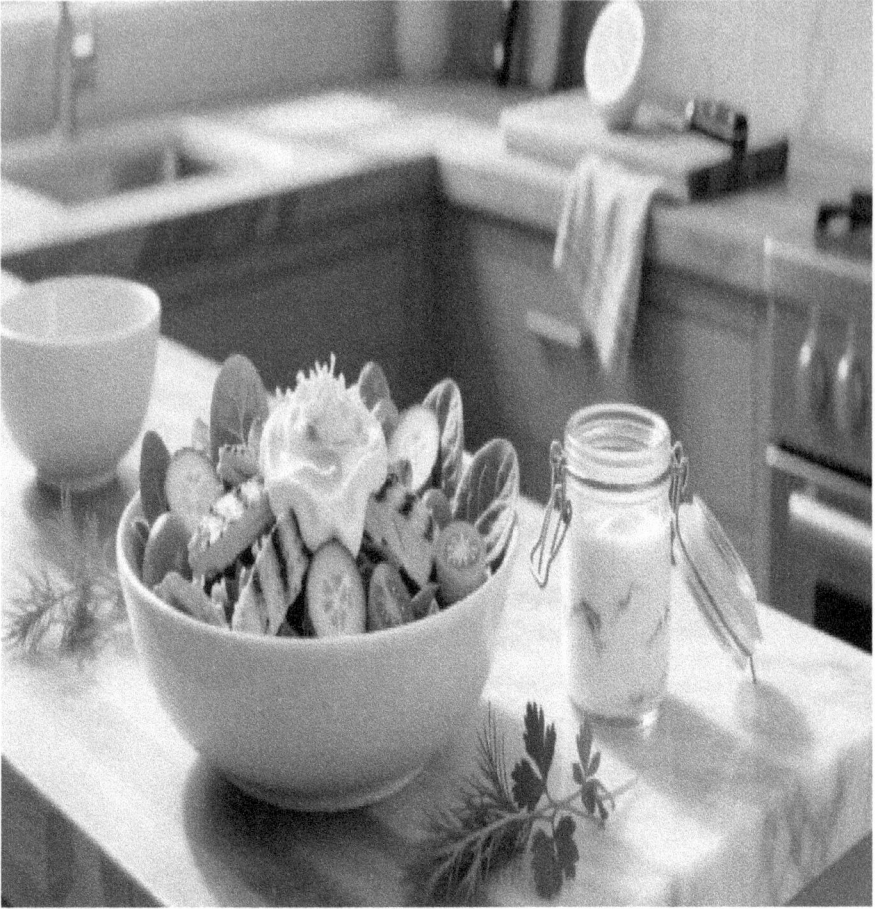

Acknowledgment

I wish to thank the countless individuals—readers, health practitioners, and nutrition experts—who have inspired this work. Your questions, insights, and shared experiences shaped this book into something practical and accessible. Above all, I am grateful to the community of everyday people seeking healthier, more energized lives; your determination proves that transformation is always possible.

www.ingramcontent.com/pod-product-compliance
Lightning Source LLC
Chambersburg PA
CBHW031131020426
42333CB00012B/325